Virtual Healing

T.S. AVINI

Virtual Healing

"Navigating the Future of Digital Healthcare"

by T.S. AVINI

Table of Contents

Chapter 1: Introduction to Digital Healthcare

In an age where a tiny computer rests comfortably in the palm of the hand, bridging continents in mere milliseconds, healthcare too is undergoing a digital revolution.

This is not merely a transformation but a reimagining of what it means to deliver and receive care. Digital healthcare, at its core, is an expansive term that encompasses a multitude of technologies designed to enhance efficiency, accuracy, and accessibility in the medical field.

Imagine a world where your smartphone not only tracks your morning run but also communicates irregularities directly to your physician in real-time.

Envision a routine where your wearable device provides a daily synopsis of your vital statistics, empowering both you and your healthcare provider with actionable insights. This is not futuristic conjecture; it is the present state of digital healthcare, evolving faster than at any other point in history.

As strange as it sounds, The impetus behind digital healthcare is multifaceted. First and foremost, there is the undeniable demand for efficiency within medical systems globally.

As populations expand and lifespans increase, healthcare systems face pressures like never before. Digital healthcare offers solutions that could alleviate some of these pressures by streamlining processes, reducing wait times, and improving patient outcomes.

Another tremendous driving force is accessibility. Traditional healthcare systems are often plagued by disparities, with rural or underserved regions suffering from a lack of access to basic medical services.

Digital technology breaks down these barriers, making healthcare more equitable. Through telemedicine, patients in remote areas can consult specialists based thousands of miles away, receiving competent care that might have otherwise been impossible.

Yet, digital healthcare is more than just technological innovation; it is a philosophical shift towards patient-centered care.

No longer passive recipients in the health narrative, patients are empowered to take charge of their wellness journeys. Mobile applications provide medication reminders, virtual reality aids in physical therapy, and personalized medicine tailors treatments to genetic profiles, all contributing to a more engaged and informed patient populace.

Many people don't realize this, but The ecosystem of digital healthcare comprises various components: electronic health records (EHRs), telemedicine, mobile health applications, wearable devices, artificial intelligence (AI), and big data.

Each of these components plays a vital role in shaping the new healthcare landscape.

EHRs, for example, have revolutionized the way medical records are stored and accessed.

Gone are the days of bulky, paper-based files that are prone to loss and misinterpretation. With just a few clicks, a patient's comprehensive medical history can be retrieved, analyzed, and shared across multiple healthcare providers, ensuring continuity and clarity in treatment plans.

Telemedicine is another cornerstone of digital healthcare, breaking down geographic barriers and offering immediate access to medical expertise.

Video consultations are not only convenient but have been proven to reduce healthcare costs and improve patient satisfaction. This modality of care becomes invaluable in circumstances such as a global pandemic, where traditional face-to-face interactions are compromised.

Mobile health, often referred to as mHealth, encompasses mobile devices and apps that provide health-related services.

The proliferation of smartphones and mobile apps has democratized health data, putting it into the hands of the people who need it the most—the patients. From tracking dietary habits and physical activity to managing chronic conditions, mHealth applications provide personalized and practical support for healthy living.

Wearable devices, such as fitness trackers and smartwatches, have inserted themselves into everyday life, doubling as motivators and monitors.

They nudge users towards healthier behaviors while providing real-time data that can be shared with healthcare providers. This constant stream of information not only offers insights into daily habits but also identifies trends that could signal potential health concerns.

Artificial Intelligence (AI) and big data analytics are perhaps the most transformative elements within digital healthcare.

AI has the capacity to analyze vast amounts of data swiftly, spotting patterns and offering predictions that might elude human practitioners. Machine learning algorithms, for instance, can aid in predictive diagnostics, offering early detection of diseases and improving treatment efficacy.

As strange as it sounds, Big data goes hand in hand with AI, as the volume of health-related data is enormous and expanding.

Together, they create opportunities for conducting research at scales previously unimaginable, revolutionizing everything from clinical trials to public health initiatives. Through the power of data, healthcare providers can not only treat but predict and prevent illness on a population scale.

While the potential of digital healthcare is immense, challenges remain.

Concerns regarding privacy and data security are paramount, as sensitive health information must be protected from breaches and unauthorized access. Moreover, the digital divide poses a risk of disenfranchisement, where certain populations—due to socioeconomic or geographic reasons—may not benefit equally from digital advancements.

As such, the transition to a digital healthcare system requires a concerted effort to address these challenges head-on.

It involves fostering an environment that prioritizes ethical standards, equitable access, and constant innovation. Policymakers, technologists, healthcare providers, and patients must collaborate to ensure that digital healthcare contributes positively to the common good without exacerbating existing disparities.

Let's not forget, The journey through digital healthcare is not a sprint but a marathon.

It demands vision, perseverance, and adaptability. As we stand on the precipice of this new age of medicine, it is essential to remain guided by the core principle that has always driven healthcare—the betterment of human life.

This book, "Virtual Healing: Navigating the Future of Digital Healthcare," invites you on a journey through the complexities and wonders of this innovative field. In the chapters to follow, we will explore each facet of digital healthcare in greater detail, examining both the opportunities and the obstacles faced by this rapidly changing world.

We will also delve into real-world examples and case studies, highlighting how technology is currently being leveraged across the globe to transform lives. Join us as we navigate the future of digital healthcare, where technology meets compassion, and innovation empowers healing.

Chapter 2: The Evolution of Telemedicine

In the not-so-distant past, the concept of seeing a doctor involved a ritual: calling the clinic to book an appointment, flipping through outdated magazines in the waiting room, and finally, the in-person interaction that often felt rushed due to the undeniable constraints on the healthcare provider's time.

Today, we stand on the cusp of a new era—telemedicine—a seismic shift that has revolutionized how healthcare services are delivered and accessed. The journey of telemedicine is a tale of innovation, driven as much by necessity as by the inexhaustible human spirit to improve and adapt.

Origins and Early Adoption

Let's not forget, Telemedicine is not a novel invention of the 21st century; its roots trace back to the mid-20th century when radio was used to provide healthcare advice to shipbound sailors.

The concept took a significant leap in the 1960s with the advent of the space race. NASA, facing the challenge of providing medical care to astronauts, developed remote medical systems that became the precursors to modern telehealth technology.

As the technology slowly seeped beyond the confines of scientific endeavors, it found its feet in rural health.

Communities isolated by geography but united by need became fertile grounds for telemedicine's early interventions. The link between remote hospitals and urban medical centers through closed-circuit television marked one of the earliest implementations, heralding a new dawn of accessibility.

Technological Advancements

In real life, Fast forward a few decades, and telemedicine underwent a technological metamorphosis driven by the digital revolution.

The proliferation of personal computers, followed by mobile technology, escalated the spread of telehealth services. Video conferencing, digital imaging, and electronic health records (EHR) grew to become cornerstones that underpinned the infrastructure of remote medical consultations.

High-speed internet further catapulted telemedicine into a new dimension, offering real-time interaction that simulated face-to-face consultations.

This became vital, particularly in specialist care, where scope and scale were often limited to urban centers. Teledermatology, telepsychiatry, and teleradiology emerged, each breaking down conventional barriers and reshaping the landscape of specialty health services.

Catalysts for Change

Let's not forget, Several factors acted as catalysts propelling telemedicine from a supplementary to a fundamental aspect of healthcare.

Rising healthcare costs, the increasing prevalence of chronic diseases, and an aging population were intrinsic pressures that demanded an efficient rethinking of medical service distribution. Telemedicine answered these calls with cost-effectiveness, expanded reach, and the ability to bring expert care to those in need rather than requiring the reverse.

Government policies and regulations, once resistant, gradually began to bend under the pressure of necessity.

Countries recognized the potential of telemedicine to bridge the healthcare gap, especially in underserved populations. Healthcare systems around the globe began to embrace telemedicine, backed by regulatory frameworks designed to address privacy, reimbursement, and licensing issues.

The Role of the Global Pandemic

Many people don't realize this, but It is impossible to discuss the evolution of telemedicine without acknowledging the role of the COVID-19 pandemic.

In early 2020, as the world grappled with the pandemic, telemedicine transitioned from a peripheral service to a central pillar of healthcare systems worldwide. In-person visits plummeted due to safety concerns, and telehealth emerged as a lifeline, maintaining continuity of care while minimizing the risk of virus transmission.

The rapid scaling of telehealth services during this period demonstrated the technology's resilience and adaptability.

Healthcare providers rapidly adapted existing systems, and new solutions sprouted almost overnight. Governments globally relaxed regulations to accommodate the burgeoning demand, and insurance companies expanded coverage for telehealth services, all of which further embedded telemedicine into the healthcare fabric.

Challenges and Barriers

Despite its rapid evolution and adoption, telemedicine faces challenges that continue to shape its trajectory.

For one, inequities in digital infrastructure create disparities in access—urban areas enjoy seamless telemedicine experiences while rural locales may struggle with internet connectivity issues. Additionally, the interplay between telemedicine and patient privacy remains a pivotal concern, necessitating robust cybersecurity measures to protect sensitive health information.

There are clinical challenges too.

Not all medical concerns can be addressed remotely, and the absence of physical examination limits diagnostic capabilities in certain cases. Consequently, telemedicine is often best used as a complement to, rather than a replacement for, traditional in-person care.

The Future of Telemedicine

Looking forward, the evolution of telemedicine promises to unlock new potentials.

Artificial Intelligence (AI) and machine learning are anticipated to augment diagnostic accuracy and personalize patient care at an unprecedented scale. Wearable devices and mobile health technologies will provide continuous health monitoring, enabling proactive interventions.

Moreover, as telemedicine becomes more ingrained in healthcare systems, the role of data will be magnified.

Aggregated data from telehealth interactions will offer insights into public health trends, guiding policy and intervention strategies.

Conclusion

Believe it or not, Telemedicine has come a long way from its experimental origins, catalyzed by technology and necessity into a sophisticated, indispensable component of modern healthcare.

As we navigate an increasingly digital future, telemedicine stands as a beacon of innovation—its evolution only beginning as we continue to embrace the future of digital healthcare.

While it may never replace the human touch that in-person care provides, telemedicine complements it uniquely.

In its continual evolution, telemedicine will undoubtedly transform how we perceive health and wellness, creating a future where healthcare isn't just reactive but inherently proactive.

Chapter 3: The Role of AI in Modern Healthcare

In the dawn of the 21st century, a monumental transformation is transpiring in the domain of healthcare, driven by the ceaseless advancement of artificial intelligence (AI). The age of digital stethoscopes and robotic surgery is not merely a glimpse into the future; it is our present reality.

Across waiting rooms, operating theaters, and research labs, AI is orchestrating a symphony of efficiencies that redefine the way healthcare is conceived and delivered. Understanding the role of AI in modern healthcare is akin to decrypting the future of human well-being itself—a future where bits and bytes are as fundamental to healing as the care of a doctor.

At the heart of AI's groundbreaking integration into healthcare is its ability to process vast quantities of data with pinpoint precision. Every instance of patient care—from an off-hand doctor's note to high-resolution imaging study—is a data point in this massive ecosystem.

Traditional healthcare methods, while effective, grapple with the sheer volume of information available. AI systems excel where human cognition is overwhelmed, effortlessly sifting through terabytes of data, discovering patterns, and producing actionable insights. This capability is not only augmentative but transformative, turning chaos into coherence.

Let's not forget, With machine learning, a branch of AI that teaches computers to learn from data without being explicitly programmed, healthcare enters an era of predictive analysis.

For instance, AI algorithms can scrutinize thousands of patient records to predict disease outbreaks, identify at-risk populations, and suggest preventive measures well before patients manifest symptoms. This prescient approach to healthcare promises not only to enhance patient outcomes but also to elevate the very standard of living by fostering proactive health measures.

Moreover, image recognition algorithms have begun revolutionizing diagnostics, particularly in fields like radiology and pathology. AI can now analyze digital scans with greater speed and accuracy than a human eye, distinguishing abnormalities from the benign at a microscopic level.

Consider a system that examines thousands of mammograms, instantly distinguishing between benign and malignant growths with accuracy that rivals the best trained specialists. This innovation doesn't replace the healthcare provider but augments their capabilities, acting as a second set of expert eyes, minimizing human error and ensuring that nothing is overlooked.

The application of AI extends beyond diagnosis and into treatment planning, providing personalized medical care. By integrating data from genetic profiles, medical history, and real-world evidence, AI systems can tailor treatments to the unique makeup of each patient.

In oncology, for instance, AI provides insights into the most effective treatment plans for cancer patients, taking into consideration genetic variations, lifestyle factors, and historical treatment outcomes. The result is personalized medicine on a scale previously unimaginable, transforming cancer care from a one-size-fits-all model to a bespoke approach.

I've seen this happen before: Telemedicine platforms empowered by AI are another leap forward, breaking barriers of time and distance, and democratizing access to healthcare. With AI-enhanced communication tools, healthcare providers can offer consultations and continuous monitoring to patients in remote regions where medical resources are scarce.

Language processing algorithms translate medical terminologies into layman's terms, ensuring that communication between provider and patient is seamless and effective. These platforms also facilitate continuous patient engagement through automated follow-ups and personalized health advice, forging a new model of patient-centric care.

In a world increasingly ravaged by systemic inequalities, AI holds promise for equitable healthcare delivery. However, as with any transformative technology, AI also presents challenges that must be addressed to harness its full potential ethically.

Issues of data privacy and consent loom large as AI systems harvest massive datasets from patients. Ensuring that data is anonymized and securely stored is paramount to maintaining trust in this digital age. Furthermore, AI models trained on biased datasets risk perpetuating existing health disparities unless intentionally adjusted through inclusive and diverse data representation.

Regulatory frameworks are evolving alongside technological advancements, striving to keep pace with the ethical intricacies posed by AI-driven healthcare.

Establishing clear guidelines that ensure AI applications are safe, effective, and equitable will be crucial in navigating the course of this digital healthcare revolution. Collaborative efforts between technologists, healthcare professionals, policymakers, and ethicists are essential to creating a cohesive ecosystem conducive to innovation while safeguarding patient well-being.

As strange as it sounds, Moreover, human touch is indispensable in the healing process. AI, while a prodigious tool, lacks the empathy intrinsic to healthcare providers.

The true value of AI lies in freeing up human caregivers from mundane tasks to focus on what they excel at—delivering compassionate, human-centered care. The integration of AI in healthcare should not lead to depersonalization but rather humanization by allowing healthcare professionals more time to engage with patients on a personal level.

As we move further into this new epoch of healthcare, the potential for AI to enhance, not replace, human capabilities appears boundless.

It is a tool for empowerment—a technological physician's assistant with a synthesis of speed, accuracy, and unfailing dedication to data. Embracing this evolution requires an open mind, a commitment to ethical standards, and a global vision where access to quality healthcare is a fundamental right for every individual.

In the warmth of hospital corridors and the sterile confines of laboratories, AI is quietly, yet profoundly, scripting a future where healthcare is not just reactive but predictive; not standard, but personalized.

The dawn of AI in healthcare is not a harbinger of a dystopian future, but rather a guiding light towards a unified vision of health that is more inclusive, efficient, and compassionate than ever before. In the tale of digital healing, AI is the pen writing new stories of hope, resilience, and the enduring human spirit.

Chapter 4: E-Health Records: Revolutionizing Patient Data

In the dawning age of digital transformation, healthcare finds itself poised at the brink of a revolution—one that is data-driven and patient-centered.

Central to this change is the emergence of electronic health records (EHRs), which promise to streamline the complexities of medical data management and redefine the patient care experience altogether. This chapter delves into the pivotal role of EHRs, charting the course forward in our journey towards optimizing digital healthcare.

The Evolution of Health Records

It's worth noting that Historically, patient information was painstakingly chronicled in paper records—bulky, susceptible to loss, and often incomplete.

The traditional model was not only inefficient but also limited in its capacity to provide a holistic view of a patient's health journey. Fast forward to today, EHRs stand as the linchpin of modern medical practice, offering seamless integration of patient information across multiple healthcare systems.

The transition from paper to pixels is more than a technological upgrade; it represents a paradigm shift towards more cohesive patient care.

EHRs enable healthcare providers to access comprehensive health records instantaneously, fostering an environment where critical data is available right at the point of care. This transformation is not just a matter of convenience but one of accuracy and life-saving potential.

Real-Time, Comprehensive Data Access

Believe it or not, One of the defining features of EHRs is the ability to provide real-time access to a plethora of patient data.

From laboratory results and imaging to medication histories and allergy alerts, EHR systems gather and present an integrated view of a patient's medical history, ensuring that healthcare professionals have all pertinent information at their fingertips. This immediacy not only expedites the decision-making process but also reduces the likelihood of human error, which has been a longstanding concern in the medical field.

Consider a scenario where a patient visits the emergency room.

With EHRs, the attending physician can quickly access the patient's past medical history, understand previous diagnoses, review current medications, and note any allergies—all without paging through stacks of paperwork or waiting for phone calls to distant clinics. This level of accessibility translates into more effective, efficient, and personalized care.

Bridging Gaps with Interoperability

It's worth noting that Interoperability—the ability of different EHR systems to communicate with each other—is crucial in crafting a unified healthcare ecosystem.

For many years, the healthcare industry grappled with siloed systems that isolated valuable patient data within individual institutions. EHRs, by their nature, aim to break down these barriers, enabling a free flow of information across diverse platforms.

In practice, interoperability can enhance collaborative care, allowing multiple healthcare providers to contribute to and access a shared patient record.

For instance, a specialist can add insights and updates to a patient's record, ensuring that the primary care physician is always in the loop. This minimizes redundant tests and procedures, ultimately reducing patient hassle and healthcare costs.

However, the challenge of achieving truly seamless interoperability remains.

Healthcare systems often utilize different software and data formats, and aligning these requires both technological and regulatory advances. Initiatives such as the Health Level Seven International (HL7) standards are already paving the way for such unification, setting a framework for data exchange across varied health information systems.

Patient Empowerment through Digital Access

The EHR revolution is not limited to healthcare providers.

Patients, too, stand to gain remarkable benefits by actively participating in their own care via EHR accessibility. Patient portals—digital platforms linked to EHRs—offer individuals a window into their own health data, empowering them to make informed decisions about their well-being.

Through these portals, patients can access their medical histories, schedule appointments, request prescription refills, and even communicate directly with their healthcare team.

This level of involvement fosters a sense of responsibility, encouraging patients to adhere to treatment plans and engage in preventive care measures.

Let's not forget, Moreover, the transparency of EHRs reassures patients of the accuracy and continuity of their care.

They can verify test results, question discrepancies, and collaborate with their doctors to tailor healthcare plans that reflect their unique needs and preferences. In essence, EHRs democratize health information, nurturing a robust partnership between patients and providers.

The Role of AI in EHR Optimization

As technology continues to evolve, artificial intelligence (AI) stands ready to enhance the efficiency and functionality of EHR systems further.

AI-powered algorithms can analyze vast datasets to detect patterns and trends, offering predictive insights that aid early diagnosis and intervention. Machine learning models, embedded within EHR systems, can suggest personalized treatment plans or flag potential drug interactions, pushing the boundaries of patient care optimization.

Believe it or not, Furthermore, natural language processing (NLP) can streamline the clinical documentation process, reducing the burden of data entry for healthcare providers.

Voice-to-text capabilities can accurately transcribe the nuances of doctor-patient interactions, generating detailed and orderly patient records. The integration of AI in EHRs not only maximizes the utility of patient data but also liberates healthcare professionals to focus on their primary mission: patient care.

Privacy and Security Concerns

While the benefits of EHRs are transformative, they are not without challenges—particularly in the realms of privacy and cybersecurity.

The wealth of data housed within EHR systems makes them attractive targets for cybercriminals, underscoring the need for stringent security measures. Ensuring the confidentiality and integrity of patient data requires robust encryption protocols, multifactor authentication, and regular security audits.

Believe it or not, Equally vital is upholding patient consent and control over their own health information.

Regulatory frameworks such as the Health Insurance Portability and Accountability Act (HIPAA) in the United States provide guidelines to protect patient privacy, but continuous vigilance and adaptation are necessary to counter emerging threats in the digital landscape. As we advance into an era of digital healthcare, establishing and maintaining trust between patients and healthcare providers is paramount.

Conclusion: Toward a Digitally Integrated Future

EHRs represent more than just a technical evolution; they symbolize the reshaping of the patient care paradigm itself.

By unlocking the potential of cohesive, real-time data access, EHRs pave the way for a future where healthcare is not only more efficient but also more personalized and proactive.

As strange as it sounds, As we stand on the precipice of this digital frontier, the challenge is to harness the full capabilities of EHRs while addressing the unique concerns they present.

By embracing innovation and maintaining a steadfast commitment to patient-centric care, we can navigate the journey toward a healthcare system that is both technologically advanced and deeply humane.

In the coming years, as EHR systems continue to evolve and adapt, they will undoubtedly serve as pivotal tools in the ongoing mission to revolutionize healthcare.

Through a synthesis of technology, collaboration, and trust, the future of digital healthcare, anchored by electronic health records, holds the promise of a healthier society, equipped and empowered to thrive amidst the rapid currents of change.

Chapter 5: Wearable Technology: The New Frontier

In the burgeoning landscape of digital healthcare, wearable technology emerges as both pioneer and protagonist, revolutionizing the way individuals monitor their health and engage with healthcare systems.

This new frontier, melding the boundaries between science and daily life, offers unprecedented opportunities for personalized care, preventative medicine, and enhanced patient engagement. Wearable devices, ranging from smartwatches to sophisticated biomonitoring systems, have transcended their initial roles as mere fitness trackers, evolving into powerful tools that capture invaluable health data in real-time.

The Evolution of Wearables

Interestingly enough, The journey of wearable technology began humbly, with devices that monitored simple metrics such as step count or sleep patterns. Over time, this sector has experienced an ideological and technological metamorphosis, integrating advanced sensors and connectivity features.

Today's wearables can track an array of physiological data, including heart rate variability, blood oxygen levels, and even electrocardiograms (ECGs). Innovations in material science and miniaturization have enabled these devices to become more accurate, less intrusive, and more accessible to the general population.

Key players such as Apple, Fitbit, and Garmin, among others, have paved the way, offering devices that not only serve as health monitors but also as lifestyle companions.

Moreover, these devices work seamlessly with smartphones and other digital platforms, stitching together a comprehensive tapestry of health data that can be shared with healthcare providers for a holistic understanding of a patient's health.

Personalized Medicine: A New Paradigm

Many people don't realize this, but At the core of wearable technology lies the promise of personalized medicine—a model of care tailored to the individual's unique health profile.

By continuously gathering data from wearables, healthcare providers can devise treatment plans that are more aligned with the individual needs of patients. Wearable devices can alert both users and their doctors to potential health issues before they become critical, shifting the paradigm from reactive to preventative care.

Imagine a scenario where a wearable device alerts a user to a potentially life-threatening arrhythmia, prompting an early visit to a healthcare provider. Early detection and intervention can significantly reduce the progression of many conditions, proving the efficacy and necessity of these tools.

Wearables also play a vital role in managing chronic conditions. Diabetic patients, for example, benefit from continuous glucose monitors, which provide real-time data, enabling them to manage their insulin levels more effectively.

Data Collection and Privacy

Believe it or not, The myriad data collected by wearables undoubtedly offer profound insights into an individual's health, but this also raises critical questions about data security and patient privacy.

As devices become more sophisticated and data transmission grows ubiquitous, ensuring the confidentiality, integrity, and availability of healthcare data becomes paramount. Moreover, tech companies and healthcare providers must work collaboratively to establish clear data governance policies, ensuring that data is handled ethically and is only accessed by authorized parties.

The standardization of health data formats and protocols is also essential to ensure interoperability across different platforms.

This requires coordinated efforts among stakeholders, including tech developers, healthcare providers, and policymakers, to ensure that the healthcare ecosystem is both secure and integrated. Achieving this balance is paramount because it builds consumer trust and enables the seamless flow of information necessary for advanced care delivery.

The Impact of AI and Machine Learning

As strange as it sounds, The integration of artificial intelligence (AI) and machine learning algorithms into wearable technology marks an exciting edge of innovation.

These technologies have the potential to analyze vast amounts of data collected by wearables, identifying patterns and generating predictive models that can forecast health outcomes. For instance, an AI-driven application could alert users about impending migraines based on historical data and environmental factors, allowing them to proactively manage the triggers and reduce severity.

Moreover, AI can facilitate personalized feedback, turning raw data into actionable insights.

This capability means that users aren't left to interpret voluminous health data alone, but instead receive clear, AI-generated guidance crafted to optimize their lifestyle and health choices. The amalgamation of wearable data and AI analysis provides a self-advancing mechanism that enhances health management capabilities continuously.

Expanding Accessibility

Interestingly enough, While wearable technology advances rapidly, there remains a pressing need to address accessibility, ensuring that these innovations benefit diverse populations.

The cost of wearables must be managed so that they do not remain the privilege of affluent users. Insurance companies and healthcare systems play crucial roles in advocating for policies and subsidies that can make wearable technology affordable and thus widely used.

Healthcare systems, particularly in developing countries, can leverage wearables to overcome infrastructural challenges and achieve broader healthcare coverage.

Remote monitoring enables clinicians to manage the health of patients in rural areas effectively, narrowing the healthcare disparity gap. Such global perspectives enable wearables to serve not just as gadgets for the tech-savvy but as transformative tools in global public health strategies.

The Human Element

In real life, Amidst the technological strides, the human element remains an indispensable ingredient in the equation.

Individuals must be educated and motivated to effectively utilize wearable technology. This education involves understanding how to interpret data, engaging with the resultant insights, and adhering to the recommended changes in lifestyle or treatment plans.

The emotional and psychological aspects of wearables also warrant consideration.

Technologies that foster user trust, enhance user experience, and integrate seamlessly into daily life have the greatest potential for impact. As wearables continue to evolve, the balance between human interaction and digital innovation will be pivotal in maintaining the effectiveness and acceptance of these technologies.

A Vision for the Future

Looking to the horizon, the future of wearable technology in digital healthcare appears boundless.

The fusion of technology and healthcare will continue to foster environments where precision medicine is not just an ambition but a reality. As innovations flourish and collaborations deepen, wearable technology will serve as a cornerstone in the vast structure of digital health—a structure that promises more engaged, informed, and healthier global citizens.

As we navigate this new frontier, the challenge lies not only in advancing technology but also in fundamentally reshaping how we envision and practice healthcare, ensuring it becomes more proactive, inclusive, and centered around the individual.

As we stride forward, wearables will lead the way—a beacon lights the path to a healthier tomorrow.

Chapter 6: Virtual Reality in Therapy and Recovery

In the ever-evolving landscape of digital healthcare, virtual reality (VR) emerges not merely as a technological marvel but as a profound source of innovation reshaping therapeutic and recovery practices.

No longer confined to the realms of gaming and entertainment, VR has breached traditional medical boundaries, offering an immersive therapeutic experience that can be transformative for both patients and practitioners alike. As we delve into the transformative potential of VR in therapy and recovery, it becomes clear that we are witnessing the dawn of a new era in healthcare.

The Immersive Path to Healing

It's worth noting that Virtual reality's prowess lies in its unparalleled ability to transport users into a meticulously crafted virtual environment that triggers a sense of presence unique to the medium. For patients undergoing therapy, this means interacting with their treatment environment in ways that were once inconceivable.

Imagine stroke patients being enveloped in an interactive world designed to facilitate neuroplasticity—where they can practice motor movements in a risk-free environment that encourages gradual progression and rewards perseverance. The immersive quality of VR allows for the simulation of real-world scenarios or entirely fantastical environments, depended on the therapeutic goals.

Furthermore, VR's capacity for personalization and adaptability in therapeutic settings cannot be overstated. Tailoring virtual environments to align with individual patient needs and preferences creates an environment uniquely suited to fostering recovery.

The spectrum of customization ranges from controlling visual and auditory stimuli to replicating specific real-world challenges the patient faces in their day-to-day life. This level of personalization not only enhances patient engagement but also fosters a sense of autonomy and control—critical components in the therapeutic journey.

Breaking Down Psychological Barriers

In real life, One of the most compelling applications of VR is in the realm of mental health treatment.

Conditions such as anxiety, PTSD, and phobias are addressed through exposure therapy—a cornerstone of cognitive behavioral therapy—which leverages VR's safe and controlled environments to present anxiety-inducing stimuli. Here, patients can confront their fears in a gradual, controlled manner, supported by their therapists who can adjust stimuli in real-time.

Consider Alex, a war veteran grappling with PTSD, haunted by memories that warp daily life into an incessant battlefield of triggers. Traditional therapy, though helpful, struggled to recreate the specificity and intensity of his experiences.

Enter VR-based exposure therapy: now, with the guidance of an astute therapist, Alex revisits those wounded places in a virtual world that mirrors past experiences yet is fundamentally safe and adjustable. Over time, this repeated exposure within a secure framework diffuses the potency of these memories, reducing PTSD's grip on daily life.

Through such applications, VR is redefining traditional therapy paradigms, offering a unique blend of realism and safety that is facilitating breakthroughs previously unachievable in conventional settings.

Revolutionizing Rehabilitation Practices

Beyond psychological therapy, the application of virtual reality in physical rehabilitation is equally groundbreaking. Traditionally, physical therapy is fraught with monotony.

The repetitive movements central to recovery can disengage patients, leading to non-compliance and protracted recovery times. Here, VR steps in as a captivating motivator—where exercises become games, and patient progress is charted in real-time, providing instant feedback and encouragement.

Take, for example, the scenario of a patient recovering from knee surgery. Engaging in VR-based therapy, the patient is no longer constrained by the physical boundaries of a rehabilitation center.

Instead, they might find themselves on serene digital mountain trails or embarking on virtual treasure hunts that incorporate prescribed movements crucial for recovery. Coupled with data-driven insights and progress tracking, this gamification not only enhances motivation but also provides therapists with invaluable analytics to refine treatment regimens over time.

Interestingly enough, VR also shines in cognitive rehabilitation, assisting patients with brain injuries or neurological disorders.

By simulating complex interactive scenarios that parallel real-world challenges, VR can improve cognitive functions such as memory, attention, and problem-solving. Patients find themselves immersed in tasks that demand active cognitive engagement, such as planning a virtual outing or solving puzzles, all tailored to rehabilitative goals.

Bridging Distances Through Telemental Health

In an era marked by global interconnectedness, VR's potential to bridge geographic and social distances is transformative. Telemental health services—providing psychiatric and psychological care at a distance—are enhancing their efficacy through VR.

In an age where mental health resources are scarce and unevenly distributed, VR provides an invaluable platform for remote therapeutic interventions. Patients in underserved areas now have access to immersive therapies spearheaded by practitioners located continents away, breaking down barriers to specialized care.

Many people don't realize this, but Moreover, in VR spaces, the formation of support networks is organically facilitated.

Virtual rehabilitation groups or therapy sessions not only elevate accountability but foster a communal atmosphere of shared experiences, breaking the isolation that so often accompanies the therapeutic journey. Patients participate in real-time group therapy sessions or peer support meetings that transcend geographical limits, expanding the therapeutic community's reach and efficacy.

Challenges on the Horizon: Navigating Ethical Boundaries

Despite the boundless promise of VR in therapeutic and recovery settings, it is crucial to negotiate its implementation thoughtfully.

The potential for overstimulation or adverse emotional reactions necessitates the establishment of rigorous ethical standards. Privacy concerns remain paramount as the immersive nature of VR captures extensive user data—compelling us to champion transparency, notarized consent, and data security.

It's worth noting that Moreover, clinicians must remain vigilant about the nuances of VR application, tailoring experiences to minimize side effects such as motion sickness or emotional discomfort.

As pioneers in this uncharted therapeutic territory, practitioners must balance enthusiasm with caution, with ongoing research spearheading the improvement of protocols and the establishment of definitive guidelines on safe usage.

Embracing the Future

As we hurtle towards a more technologically integrated future, virtual reality stands as a beacon of innovation that promises to elevate therapeutic experiences profoundly.

For patients, VR translates dreams of rehabilitation to realms beyond imagination—where progress is palpable and personalized, each session a step closer to healing. For practitioners, it embodies a dynamic tool that enriches the therapeutic repertoire and augments traditional methodologies with revolutionary precision and limitless potential.

In this digital age, the convergence of technology and therapy redefines boundaries, illuminating the healing path with vibrant landscapes of virtual possibilities.

As VR continues to evolve, we stand at the precipice of a dramatic shift in healthcare—one where realities are as virtual as they are healing. Embrace it, for the future of recovery is beautifully immersive.

Chapter 7: AI-Driven Diagnostics: A New Paradigm

In recent years, a subtle yet profound transformation has been sweeping through the corridors of healthcare systems worldwide. The force behind this shift is not a new wonder drug or a groundbreaking surgical technique; rather, it is rooted in the digital realm—as unassuming algorithms power a dynamic transformation.

Artificial intelligence, once the stuff of science fiction, is now reshaping healthcare diagnostics in ways that were unimaginable a few decades ago. This chapter delves into this new paradigm, exploring how AI-driven diagnostics are revolutionizing the practice of medicine and the promise they hold for the future.

The Evolution of Diagnostics

To fully appreciate the impact of AI in diagnostics, we must first understand the evolution of medical diagnostics.

Traditionally, the role of diagnostics has been the purview of skilled clinicians, reliant on years of training and experience to interpret patient symptoms, imaging, and laboratory tests. Diagnostic processes often involved time-consuming manual analysis, subject to the variability of human judgment and the breadth of individual experience.

In contrast, AI brings to the table an unprecedented capacity for data analysis and pattern recognition.

At its core, AI-driven diagnostics leverage machine learning algorithms to identify subtleties in medical data that might elude even the most observant clinician. With the ability to process vast amounts of information quickly and accurately, AI not only enhances the precision of diagnoses but also promises a democratization of healthcare access, as these technologies become more widely available.

The Mechanics of AI Diagnostics

Believe it or not, Artificial intelligence in diagnostics operates through a framework built on data—and lots of it.

Machine learning, a subset of AI, utilizes historical data to train algorithms, teaching them to recognize patterns and correlations that are indicative of specific diseases or conditions. For instance, AI systems can be trained on millions of medical images to accurately differentiate between benign and malignant tumors.

One of the most well-known applications is in radiology, where AI algorithms are used to analyze X-rays, CT scans, and MRIs.

Trained to detect anomalies as minute as a few pixels, these algorithms can identify early signs of diseases like cancer, thereby enabling earlier interventions. This not only improves patient outcomes but dramatically increases the efficiency of healthcare systems by streamlining the diagnostic process.

Moreover, AI thrives in environments with big data.

One critical advantage is its ability to integrate and analyze disparate datasets—combining electronic health records, genomic information, and lifestyle data—to offer a more comprehensive assessment of a patient's health. This integrative approach allows for personalized diagnostics, tailoring healthcare solutions to the unique genetic and environmental factors affecting each individual patient.

Practical Applications and Success Stories

Across the globe, AI is driving diagnostic innovation in powerful ways.

In the UK, the National Health Service (NHS) has partnered with technology companies to implement AI in routine diagnostic workflows, particularly in cancer diagnostics. These AI systems have exhibited remarkable success rates, sometimes outperforming human radiologists in identifying early cancer indicators.

In the United States, healthcare providers like Mayo Clinic and Cleveland Clinic are integrating AI systems that aid in disease detection and management.

At Mayo Clinic, AI algorithms are instrumental in analyzing cardiac images, leading to more accurate diagnoses of heart conditions. Similarly, Cleveland Clinic is utilizing AI to predict patient outcomes based on complex data inputs, enabling more effective treatment planning.

Globally, AI-driven platforms such as Google DeepMind are pushing boundaries with programs like DeepMind Health.

Known for its development of AlphaGo, an AI program that defeated a world champion Go player, DeepMind now turns its attention to diagnostics—developing AI systems capable of predicting eye diseases by analyzing retinal scans with extraordinary precision.

Challenges and Ethical Considerations

While the potential of AI-driven diagnostics is immense, this new paradigm is not without its challenges.

Data privacy remains a paramount concern, as AI systems must access sensitive patient information to function effectively. Ensuring proper data security measures are in place is crucial to maintaining patient trust and complying with regulations such as the General Data Protection Regulation (GDPR) in Europe.

Many people don't realize this, but Another ethical consideration is the potential displacement of healthcare jobs.

As AI assumes greater responsibilities in diagnostics, there are fears that the role of human diagnosticians may diminish. However, many experts argue for a collaborative model, where AI acts as an augmentative tool that enhances, rather than replaces, human expertise.

Transparency and interpretability of AI algorithms also present significant challenges.

In medical diagnostics, understanding how an AI system arrives at a particular conclusion is critical for validation and trust. Efforts are being made to develop explainable AI, ensuring that the decision-making processes are transparent and comprehensible to healthcare professionals.

The Future Landscape of AI-Driven Diagnostics

Looking ahead, the future of AI diagnostics appears buoyant with promise.

Continuous advancements in AI technology will further bolster its capabilities, offering even more accurate, faster, and scalable diagnostic solutions. The growing repository of global health data will refine AI algorithms, making them smarter and more adaptable to a multitude of healthcare challenges.

Furthermore, the integration of AI with other emerging technologies—such as wearable devices and telemedicine—stands to redefine patient monitoring and disease management.

Imagine a future where a simple smartphone app, powered by AI, alerts individuals to potential health risks before they manifest into serious conditions. Such innovations will empower patients, offering proactive rather than reactive healthcare.

In conclusion, AI-driven diagnostics represent a new paradigm in digital healthcare—one that is set to transform the landscape of medicine.

By harnessing the power of artificial intelligence, we can achieve a future where accurate, timely, and personalized diagnostic information is accessible to all, revolutionizing the way we understand and manage health. As we navigate this transformative journey, it is vital to remain vigilant about ethical considerations, ensuring these technologies serve to enhance human health and well-being.

Chapter 8: The Rise of Health Apps

In an era where our phones seldom stray far from our hands, they have evolved from devices of mere communication to gateways of endless possibilities. Among these possibilities lies a profound transformation in healthcare: the rise of health apps.

Health apps are the vanguard of the digital health revolution, bridging the gap between traditional healthcare services and the demands of a tech-savvy generation. This chapter delves into the multifaceted world of health apps, examining their impact, opportunities, and the challenges they present as we navigate the future of digital healthcare.

The journey of health apps began humbly, with rudimentary applications that tracked physical activity and provided basic health information.

Today, they are intricate and sophisticated platforms capable of delivering personalized health advice, real-time monitoring, and comprehensive management of chronic conditions. Health apps now form an ecosystem that encompasses wellness, fitness, medical reference, diagnostic, clinical, and even mental health services.

The accessibility of health apps is one of their most compelling attributes. With a global population that increasingly leans on smartphones, health apps offer access to healthcare for those in remote and underserved areas.

They empower individuals by placing health management tools right at their fingertips, quite literally democratizing healthcare. Patients no longer need to travel long distances or endure lengthy waits for routine consultations. Instead, they can engage in virtual visits with healthcare providers, access their medical records, and even participate in mental health therapies — all from their smartphones.

A tremendous asset of health apps is their ability to encourage preventive care. By sending reminders for vaccinations, screenings, and medications, as well as offering daily wellness tips, these apps foster a culture of proactive health management.

This supports the global health agenda of reducing the incidence of preventable diseases and conditions. The potential for predictive analytics, harnessed through vast quantities of user-generated data, offers a promising horizon where health apps not only track existing conditions but anticipate developing health issues, affording early intervention.

Consider the app that provides diabetic patients with real-time glucose monitoring integrated with their nutrition plans. This level of personalization allows for dynamic, tailored healthcare solutions.

Patients can adjust their diets and exercise regimes based on accurate metrics, preventing complications and truly becoming partners in their health journey. For patients with chronic illnesses, health apps can deliver comprehensive care plans, sending alerts about necessary lifestyle changes and enabling ongoing communication with healthcare professionals — all while compiling an invaluable record of patient data.

At first glance, Moreover, mental health applications have seen a significant uptrend in both usage and availability.

These apps offer tools for meditation, stress management, and cognitive Behavioral Therapy (CBT), providing support that was once restricted to clinician's offices. As the stigma surrounding mental illness begins to lift, more users feel comfortable accessing these apps, finding solace in guided meditation, and forming supportive virtual communities where they can share experiences and seek advice.

However, as much as health apps offer undeniable advantages, they are not without their challenges. Notably, issues around data privacy and security loom large.

With healthcare data being particularly sensitive, users are rightly concerned about how their data is collected, stored, and used. Breaches could have severe implications not only for personal privacy but also for trust in the digital health landscape. Thus, developers are tasked with implementing robust security protocols and transparent data policies to safeguard user information.

Another hurdle in the widespread adoption of health apps is ensuring their effectiveness and reliability. With an overwhelming number of apps available, the quality and accuracy of the content can vary drastically.

To navigate this challenge, regulatory bodies have started establishing guidelines for health apps, beginning to subject them to rigorous testing much like traditional medical devices. Collaborations between app developers, healthcare professionals, and regulatory agencies are essential to ensure that these digital tools deliver credible and effective healthcare solutions.

To be honest, Interoperability also stands as a critical issue.

Health apps must seamlessly integrate with existing electronic health records (EHR) systems and other digital health frameworks. Achieving this integration requires standardized data formats and communication protocols, fostering a digital healthcare ecosystem where information flows effortlessly and securely between apps, healthcare providers, and patients.

Looking forward, artificial intelligence (AI) stands poised to revolutionize health apps further.

By building AI-driven algorithms into apps, developers can enhance diagnostic capabilities, personalize treatment recommendations, and predict health outcomes with unprecedented accuracy. Language processing technologies can further break down barriers by offering multilingual support, making health apps accessible to diverse demographics across the globe.

As we stand at the cusp of a digital healthcare renaissance, health apps represent both a promise and a puzzle. They promise a future where healthcare is more patient-centric, accessible, and efficient.

Simultaneously, they challenge the boundaries of our current healthcare models, urging us to rethink data security, regulation, and interoperability. As consumers, developers, and healthcare professionals continue to explore these digital frontiers, one thing is certain: health apps are not just an adjunct to our health systems—they are integral to envisioning and forging the future of healthcare.

Believe it or not, In this rapidly evolving space, one might wonder: what comes next? Perhaps it will be an era where our wearables and phones communicate seamlessly with public health infrastructures, where health apps become not just personal assistants but integral facets of population health management.

The key lies not only in the technology itself, but in how we choose to wield it, ensuring that the rise of health apps leads to a healthier, more equitable world for all.

Chapter 9: Robotics in Surgery and Rehabilitation

In the grand tapestry of human history, few innovations have had the transformative impact on healthcare that robotics in surgery and rehabilitation are currently wielding.

As we peer into the future of medicine, we envision not just the potential for enhanced precision and effectiveness, but a profound redefinition of what it means to heal and to be healed.

The integration of robotics into surgical procedures is not just about machinery; it is a harmonious blend of cutting-edge technology and human expertise.

Robotic-assisted surgery represents the confluence of intricate engineering and advanced surgical skill, offering a glimpse into an era of unparalleled precision. Where once surgeons relied solely upon their hands to execute complex maneuvers, robotic systems now enhance their capabilities, providing tools that move with millimeter precision and steadiness beyond human physiology.

Many people don't realize this, but Consider the da Vinci Surgical System, a veritable pioneer in robotic-assisted surgery.

It provides surgeons with 3D high-definition visualization and magnification of the surgical site, while the robotic arms translate the surgeon's hand movements into smaller, more precise actions within the patient's body. This enhanced visibility and precision can significantly reduce recovery times, minimize surgical trauma, and enhance the overall outcome for patients.

Yet, as wondrous as these machines are, they do not operate independently. Instead, they augment the surgeon's abilities, serving as extensions of their hands, guided by clinical judgment and expertise.

Critics once feared that such technologies would distance caregivers from patients, yet they have found the opposite to be true. The precision of robotic surgery often allows for less invasive techniques, reducing patient recovery times and allowing caregivers to focus more on post-operative care and rehabilitation.

Beyond the confines of the operating room, robotics is redefining rehabilitation. In the aftermath of surgery or severe injury, rehabilitation is where the true healing journey begins.

The incorporation of robotics into physical therapy has transformed it into a dynamic process, adapting exercises in real-time to respond to the patient's progress. Through sophisticated sensors and algorithms, these devices provide data-driven insights into the patient's improvement over time, allowing therapists to tailor programs with unmatched specificity.

At first glance, Take for instance robotic exoskeletons.

These devices, once relegated to the realm of science fiction, are now revolutionizing physical therapy for conditions ranging from spinal cord injuries to stroke recovery. By supporting and guiding limbs through a range of motion, robotic exoskeletons can help patients relearn motor skills and regain strength with greater efficiency.

Furthermore, the repetitive precision that robotics offers can accelerate the healing process.

Unlike human therapists who may tire over time, robotic systems maintain consistent delivery of therapy, ensuring that each session is as effective as the last. This technology also empowers patients, allowing them to engage in intensive rehabilitation sessions autonomously and with confidence.

However, the road to widespread implementation is not without its hurdles. Technical mastery of these systems requires rigorous training, while ethical considerations must be addressed.

With robots providing more autonomous actions, questions about accountability and patient safety inevitably arise. We must tread carefully, ensuring that the integration of robotics is driven by patient welfare rather than technological novelty.

In real life, Moreover, the costs associated with robotic systems are non-trivial.

While the long-term benefits such as reduced rehospitalization and expedited recovery can offset initial outlays, the significant up-front investment remains a barrier for many healthcare facilities, particularly in underserved regions.

To overcome these challenges, collaboration is key.

Cross-disciplinary partnerships between engineers, clinicians, and policymakers are essential to drive innovation, reduce costs, and develop equitable models of care. Furthermore, ongoing research is critical to refine and expand the applications of robotics within healthcare, maximizing its potential to transform lives.

The evolving field of robotics in surgery and rehabilitation underscores an essential truth: the future of healthcare lies not in replacing the human touch but augmenting it.

By leveraging the precision of robotic systems, the empathy of caregivers, and the resilience of patients, we stand on the cusp of a new era in healing.

Believe it or not, In this light, the journey of integrating robotics into healthcare is both a technical quest and a profoundly human one.

It challenges us to envision a future where machines serve as partners in care, empowering healthcare professionals and enhancing the lives of patients.

As we continue to innovate and explore the possibilities, one thing remains clear: robotics in surgery and rehabilitation promises not just to reshape the healthcare landscape but to redefine what is possible in the art and science of healing.

Whether on the threshold of the operating room or the path to recovery, robotics offers a future where the line between human and machine blurs, and healing is no longer bound by limitations.

Chapter 10: Blockchain for Securing Health Information

In an era where digital transformation is redefining every aspect of our lives, healthcare stands at the precipice of a major revolution.

The emergence of blockchain technology heralds a transformative shift in how health information is secured, shared, and utilized, offering unparalleled opportunities to enhance privacy, security, and interoperability in healthcare systems.

When it comes to sensitive health information, security is paramount.

The traditional centralized databases used in healthcare systems are susceptible to a range of threats, from data breaches to unauthorized access. Enter blockchain—a distributed ledger technology that promises to safeguard health information with unprecedented levels of trust and transparency.

Understanding Blockchain in Healthcare

At its core, blockchain is a decentralized ledger that records transactions across multiple computers so that the recorded information cannot be altered retroactively.

This technology ensures that every participant in the network has access to the same data, providing a single source of truth that is both transparent and immutable.

In healthcare, blockchain can be harnessed to create robust frameworks for managing electronic health records (EHRs).

Imagine a world where your health data is not confined to any single provider's server but is instead shared seamlessly, with your permission, across your entire network of care providers. Blockchain facilitates a secure and private exchange of health data, enhancing both patient care and operational efficiency.

Securing Health Information with Blockchain

One of the foremost advantages of blockchain in securing health information is its fundamentally decentralized nature.

Unlike traditional databases susceptible to single-point failures, a blockchain-based approach distributes data across a vast network of nodes. This decentralization makes hacking attempts considerably more challenging, as an attacker would need to compromise a majority of the nodes simultaneously to alter the data.

Moreover, blockchain employs cryptographic techniques to ensure that the data being stored is tamper-proof.

Each block in the chain is linked to the preceding one, and each transaction within the block is secured via encryption. This means any attempt to alter one block would require altering every subsequent block—an effort that is practically infeasible with current technology.

Patient Empowerment and Data Privacy

Blockchain offers a paradigm shift in how patients interact with their health information.

Traditionally, patients have had limited access to their health data, often stored in silos across various healthcare institutions. Blockchain changes this dynamic by positioning patients at the center of their own health data universe.

With blockchain, patients can grant or revoke access to their records with precision, allowing specific providers access to only relevant portions of their health information.

This granular level of control empowers patients, fostering a new era of patient autonomy and engagement in their healthcare journeys.

Additionally, blockchain's inherent transparency means that patients can always see who accessed their records and when ensuring that there is clear accountability and reducing the potential for unauthorized data use.

Interoperability and Efficiency

Interoperability—the ability to share and interpret data across disparate systems—is a critical challenge in modern healthcare.

Blockchains can significantly enhance interoperability by serving as a universal language through which disparate EHR systems can communicate effectively and securely.

As strange as it sounds, This enhanced interoperability translates to greater efficiency in the healthcare system.

By alleviating administrative burdens and reducing duplication of tests and procedures, blockchain can potentially cut costs and expedite patient care. Moreover, the ability to have real-time access to comprehensive patient data can greatly enhance decision-making and lead to improved health outcomes.

Challenges and Considerations

While the potential of blockchain technology in healthcare is enormous, it is not without its challenges. First and foremost, there is the issue of scalability.

The current capacity of blockchain networks to handle the volume of transactions in large, complex healthcare environments is limited. Ongoing research and innovation are needed to develop scalable blockchain frameworks that can meet the demands of the sector.

As strange as it sounds, Moreover, data privacy in blockchain must be carefully managed.

While the transparency of the blockchain is one of its strengths, maintaining patient confidentiality is crucial. Hence, healthcare-specific blockchain applications must employ advanced encryption and anonymization techniques to protect sensitive patient data.

Another consideration is the integration of blockchain solutions with existing healthcare systems, which can be resource-intensive and necessitates alignment with regulatory standards such as HIPAA and GDPR.

It requires collaboration across technology developers, healthcare providers, and regulators to develop standards and protocols that ensure compliance while leveraging blockchain's potential.

Future Prospects

The future of blockchain in healthcare looks promising.

There are myriad potential applications beyond just securing health records—from streamlining clinical trials to drug supply chain verification, and even personalized medicine. As blockchain matures and overcomes current challenges, it will likely become a foundational technology in the digital healthcare landscape.

In conclusion, blockchain offers a powerful tool for securing health information, positioning patients at the center of their care, and facilitating a more efficient, interoperable healthcare system.

Its implementation, while complex, promises to transform how we manage and protect the most sensitive information we possess—our health records. As we venture further into the digital age, the integration of innovative technologies like blockchain into healthcare systems is not simply a possibility but a necessity for creating a resilient, secure, and patient-centric healthcare ecosystem.

Chapter 11: Personalized Medicine: The Genomic Revolution

In a quiet corner of a bustling city hospital, a patient sits anxiously, awaiting the results of a genetic test.

Moments later, a doctor enters the room, carrying a tablet that holds not just a diagnosis, but a blueprint—a highly personalized treatment plan tailored uniquely to the individual's genetic makeup. This scene, which once belonged to the realm of science fiction, is rapidly becoming commonplace in the age of the genomic revolution.

The concept of personalized medicine has been around for decades, but it was the sequencing of the human genome at the turn of the millennium that truly ignited a transformation in healthcare.

Once considered the exclusive province of the future, the power to tailor medical treatment to the individual based on their genetic profile is now within our grasp, ushering in a new era of possibilities and challenges.

To grasp the potential of personalized medicine, one must understand the interplay of genes and health.

The human genome, akin to a vast instruction manual, dictates the body's functions, vulnerabilities, and strengths. Each human being carries a unique set of about 20,000-25,000 genes, resulting in variations that influence susceptibility to diseases, response to medications, and overall health.

The genomic revolution has turned these genetic blueprints into actionable medical insights.

Advances in technology have made genetic testing faster, cheaper, and more accessible than ever before. As a result, healthcare providers can now delve into individual genetic data to uncover predispositions to certain conditions and devise preventive strategies or interventions well before symptoms manifest.

Consider, for instance, the treatment of cancer—an area where personalized medicine has already made significant inroads. Traditional cancer therapies often involve one-size-fits-all approaches: chemotherapy, radiation, surgery.

However, these methods do not account for the genetic diversity in tumor profiles. Personalized medicine, in contrast, leverages genomic data to identify specific mutations driving cancer growth in an individual patient. With this information, targeted therapies can be developed to precisely attack the malignant cells while sparing healthy tissue, thus minimizing side effects and enhancing treatment efficacy.

To be honest, Beyond oncology, the implications of personalized medicine span nearly every branch of healthcare. Cardiovascular diseases, where genetic factors play a substantial role, stand to be particularly impacted.

Identifying key genetic variations can lead to the early detection of potential heart issues, allowing for proactive measures such as lifestyle changes or targeted medications. This preemptive approach not only improves quality of life but reduces the financial burden on healthcare systems with preventive care outweighing costly treatments.

Furthermore, personalized medicine addresses a critical problem in pharmacology: variability in drug response.

It has been widely observed that medications effective for some can be ineffective or even harmful to others due to genetic differences. Pharmacogenomics, a subset of personalized medicine, aims to solve this conundrum by utilizing genetic data to predict how a patient will respond to a specific drug, significantly reducing the trial-and-error methods prevalent in current treatments.

However, the path to widespread adoption of personalized medicine is not without hurdles. Ethical considerations loom large given the sensitive nature of genetic data.

Safeguarding this information becomes paramount to prevent misuse, discrimination, or breaches of privacy. This calls for robust regulatory frameworks and secure data handling practices to protect individuals' rights while fostering innovation.

Moreover, the integration of personalized medicine into existing healthcare structures demands significant adaptation.

Healthcare providers must update their training and practice to incorporate genomic information into patient care effectively. This transformation also requires collaboration across various disciplines—geneticists, bioinformaticians, clinicians, and policymakers—to navigate the complexities of interpreting genetic data and translating it into clinical applications.

Education plays a crucial role in empowering patients to embrace personalized medicine.

Demystifying genetic data and explaining its implications to patients enriches their engagement in care decisions. A well-informed patient is better equipped to understand the significance of genetic predispositions and the rationale behind personalized therapeutic strategies, fostering a collaborative physician-patient relationship.

The economic landscape of personalized medicine is another area ripe for exploration.

As costs of genomic sequencing decrease, the potential to democratize access grows, yet equitable availability remains a concern. Strategic models must be developed to ensure that advancements do not cater solely to affluent populations but are instead integrated into public health services, broadening their reach and impact.

Let's not forget, In conclusion, the genomic revolution represents a seismic shift in the landscape of medicine. Personalized medicine, grounded in the understanding of genetic blueprints, heralds a future where healthcare is both predictive and precise, catering to the individual rather than relying on approximations.

While challenges remain, the potential benefits of this approach—ranging from enhanced treatment outcomes to preventive care—underscore the importance of continued investment and collaboration in this burgeoning field. As we navigate the future of digital healthcare, personalized medicine stands as a beacon of hope, illuminating pathways to longer, healthier lives for all.

Chapter 12: Telehealth in Rural and Underserved Areas

In the sprawling canvas of digital transformation, telehealth stands as one of its most revolutionary brushstrokes.

Its emergence is not merely about technological advancement; it's a profound reimagining of healthcare delivery, particularly for rural and underserved areas. This chapter explores how telehealth is bridging the gap, bringing healthcare to doorsteps that were once, metaphorically and literally, miles away.

The Geography of Access

Let's not forget, Rural and underserved areas have historically faced challenges in accessing quality healthcare. The geographical expanse, limited infrastructure, and scarcity of healthcare professionals have compounded into a formidable barrier.

Enter telehealth. With the advent of virtual care technologies, these regions are seeing a seismic shift in healthcare accessibility. Medical consultations, follow-ups, and even specialized services that required arduous travels are now possible from a simple, digital interface.

Telehealth leverages video calls, remote monitoring, and mobile health apps to extend the reach of healthcare services beyond the bounds of traditional clinics.

Patients can connect with healthcare providers in real-time, reducing the need for travel and minimizing the disruption of everyday life. The immediacy of care is enhanced, and with it, the potential for earlier diagnosis and intervention.

The Technological Bridge

As strange as it sounds, Technology is often viewed as a privilege of the urban and affluent, yet its democratizing potential is most vividly demonstrated in how telehealth operates in rural areas. The primary challenge—one of digital infrastructure—is being addressed with concerted efforts to increase broadband connectivity.

Initiatives spearheaded by governments and private enterprises are slowly but surely stitching a web of connectivity across remote landscapes. Satellite internet, fiber optics, and mobile broadband are the threads that interweave this digital fabric, supporting the tapestry of virtual healthcare.

The advent of 5G technology promises to further revolutionize this, offering faster data speeds and more reliable connectivity.

For the farmers, ranchers, and residents of distant hamlets, this means consulting specialists and receiving medical advice without the physical journey.

Telehealth platforms are increasingly designed to be user-friendly, with interfaces that account for low-tech proficiency and language barriers, further personalizing the healthcare experience.

A New Paradigm of Care

As strange as it sounds, Telehealth is not just about convenience; it's about transforming paradigms of care. It introduces a model that accommodates the unique lifestyles and needs of rural communities.

For example, agricultural cycles often dictate availability; telehealth provides the flexibility for healthcare to adapt to such rhythms. This adaptability is crucial in maintaining continuity of care, particularly for chronic conditions that require regular monitoring and management.

Imagine a chronic diabetes patient living miles away from the nearest health facility.

Regular check-ins usually necessitate taking off work, which in a rural setting can have significant economic and personal repercussions. However, through telehealth, the same patient can use a smartphone or a computer to consult with healthcare professionals, share glucose readings, and adjust treatment plans without leaving home.

Challenges and Opportunities

To be honest, Despite its promise, the integration of telehealth in rural and underserved areas is not without challenges.

The digital divide remains a substantive hurdle, with areas lacking reliable internet access still at risk of being left behind. Efforts to improve infrastructure must therefore be not just consistent but also innovative, incorporating community-based solutions and input.

Data privacy and security present another layer of complexity. While urban centers might have advanced cybersecurity measures, rural communities often lack similar protections.

Building trust is crucial—patients need assurance that their personal health information is secure. Legislation and regulations must also evolve in tandem with technological innovations to safeguard users and facilitate seamless cross-border care.

However, the beauty of telehealth lies in its ability to not only face these challenges but also to turn them into opportunities for further innovation.

It encourages the healthcare ecosystem to think locally yet act digitally, considering the socio-cultural nuances that define each community.

Community Involvement and Empowerment

A successful telehealth strategy in rural and underserved regions hinges on community involvement.

Solutions that are co-created with input from local residents stand a better chance of being adopted and sustained. Local champions and health workers, well-versed in the cultural and linguistic context, play a critical role in educating and aligning health practices with digital platforms.

Moreover, telehealth can empower these communities by decentralizing healthcare knowledge.

With resources and educational tools digitized, health literacy can improve, empowering individuals to take an active role in their well-being. This ripple effect can contribute to healthier populations and, over time, reduce the burden on healthcare systems.

Conclusion: Crafting a Connected Future

In crafting a digitally connected future, telehealth is not just an option for rural and underserved areas—it is an essential ingredient.

At its core, telehealth embodies the principle that healthcare is a right, not a privilege defined by ZIP codes or mileage markers.

As we stand on the precipice of an increasingly digitized world, the responsibility lies in ensuring that these technological advancements contribute to closing gaps rather than widening them.

The road ahead, though lined with obstacles, is illuminated by potential—the potential to weave technology, empathy, and innovation into a tapestry of accessible healthcare for all.

Believe it or not, In embracing this paradigm, we are not just transforming how healthcare is delivered; we are fostering a future where geography no longer defines destiny.

This future, powered by telehealth, holds the promise of bringing quality care to every corner, every community, and every individual, aligned with the belief that where you live should not determine the care you receive.

Chapter 13: Mental Health and Digital Therapeutics

In the ever-evolving landscape of digital healthcare, a profound transformation is underway, redefining how we approach mental health.

The burgeoning field of digital therapeutics is not just a glimpse into the future; it is an active force reshaping our present. As we venture into this brave new world, we find ourselves at a crossroads of technology and empathy, where the promise of digital tools is measured by their ability to heal the human mind.

At its core, digital therapeutics for mental health expands beyond mere convenience.

These innovations are designed with precision, aiming to provide accessible, personalized, and effective care to millions grappling with mental health challenges. Harnessing the power of data analytics, artificial intelligence, and digital platforms, these tools usher in a paradigm shift in how treatment is delivered and experienced.

Navigating Accessibility and Stigma

One of the most formidable barriers in mental healthcare has always been accessibility. Physical distance, limited resources, and the societal stigma surrounding mental illness have often obstructed individuals from seeking help.

Digital therapeutics, however, offer a transformative solution by breaking down these barriers. Consider the smartphone in your pocket. It is no longer just a device for communication; it is a portal to healthcare.

Teletherapy platforms, for instance, provide immediate access to licensed therapists, enabling individuals to receive professional help from the comfort of their own homes.

This not only reduces the stigma associated with visiting a mental health clinic but also allows those in remote or underserved areas to seek care that might otherwise be out of reach. In a world where time and distance are often the adversaries of well-being, digital therapeutics are rendering these obstacles obsolete.

Personalization Through Precision

Yet, the promise of digital therapeutics goes beyond accessibility. Perhaps their most revolutionary aspect is the ability to personalize treatment with unprecedented precision.

Imagine a therapy regimen tailored specifically to your unique psychological profile, lifestyle, and preferences. This is where artificial intelligence comes into play, analyzing vast datasets to develop bespoke treatment plans.

Consider mobile applications designed to support mental health. These platforms utilize machine learning algorithms to track mood patterns, identify triggers, and offer coping strategies tailored to the individual.

They bridge the gap between traditional therapy and self-care, empowering users to take control of their mental health journey. The algorithms become companions, learning and adapting to the user's needs, offering insights that were previously hidden.

Gamification and Engagement

In the quest to make mental health treatment more engaging, the concept of gamification emerges as an innovative ally.

Gamification, the integration of game elements into non-game contexts, is transforming how therapeutic interventions are delivered. By incorporating rewards, challenges, and interactive elements, digital therapeutics are making the path to mental wellness more engaging and less daunting.

Consider a digital platform designed to help users manage anxiety.

This platform might present relaxation exercises formatted as levels in a game, where users earn rewards for completing meditation sessions or reaching relaxation milestones. Such gamified elements not only motivate individuals to stick to their therapeutic regimen but also transform the often overwhelming journey of mental health recovery into an enjoyable and rewarding experience.

Ethical Considerations and Privacy Concerns

In the pursuit of innovation, it is crucial to navigate ethical considerations with diligence. The collection and analysis of personal data are integral to the functioning of digital therapeutics.

However, they also raise valid concerns about privacy and data security. As we embrace this digital frontier, it is imperative that robust safeguards are implemented to protect sensitive information.

Transparency in data usage, informed consent, and stringent security measures must be prioritized to maintain the delicate balance between innovation and privacy.

Users must feel confident that their personal information is treated with the utmost care and respect. Collaboration between technologists, healthcare professionals, and policymakers is paramount to establish ethical standards that safeguard the rights of every individual engaging with digital therapeutics.

Fostering Human Connection

While digital therapeutics offer a wealth of opportunities, they should not be perceived as a replacement for human connection but rather as an enhancement.

The role of empathetic communication, understanding, and face-to-face interaction remains invaluable in mental health care. Digital tools should complement the human touch, augmenting the capacity of healthcare professionals to provide compassionate care.

Consider virtual support groups facilitated through digital platforms.

These spaces bring individuals together, offering a sense of community and shared experience that is vital for those facing similar challenges. Here, the digital world meets the human need for connection, creating supportive environments where individuals can share stories, offer encouragement, and foster meaningful relationships.

Looking Ahead

As we stand on the cusp of this digital revolution in mental health care, the potential of digital therapeutics is both exhilarating and profound.

The convergence of technology and mental well-being holds the promise of a more inclusive, personalized, and effective approach to treatment. Yet, the journey is just beginning, and it invites continuous exploration, innovation, and ethical vigilance.

In embracing the possibilities of digital therapeutics, we have the opportunity to rewrite the narrative of mental health care. Through collaboration, empathy, and technological ingenuity, we can create a future where mental wellness is within reach for everyone, irrespective of their circumstances.

The digital therapeutic revolution beckons us to imagine, innovate, and heal in ways that were once only the realm of imagination. In this landscape, the human mind finds a resilient ally in the digital realm, and together, they navigate the path toward healing and hope.

Chapter 14: The Ethics of Digital Healthcare

In the age of rapid technological advancement, digital healthcare emerges as both a promise and a challenge.

It offers unprecedented opportunities to improve access, efficiency, and effectiveness but also poses complex ethical questions that require careful consideration. As we stand at the crossroads of this digital healthcare revolution, it is crucial to navigate its ethical landscape with precision and foresight.

The integration of digital technologies in healthcare is transforming traditional paradigms of patient care.

From telemedicine to wearable health trackers, artificial intelligence (AI) diagnostics to personalized medicine, these innovations promise to enhance patient outcomes and democratize healthcare access. However, they also raise ethical concerns that we must address to ensure a fair, just, and humane healthcare system.

It's worth noting that Foremost among these concerns is privacy. In the digital age, patient information is increasingly stored, processed, and shared across various platforms, often without explicit consent or transparency.

The question of who owns this information and how it can be used is a contentious issue. Patients must have the right to control their data and be assured that it is secure and used ethically. The risk of data breaches and unauthorized access to personal health records is a significant concern, necessitating robust cybersecurity measures and clear regulatory frameworks.

Beyond privacy, the issue of equity is paramount. While digital healthcare has the potential to bridge gaps in access to services, it also risks widening disparities.

Not everyone has equal access to digital technology, and socio-economic, geographical, and generational divides must be addressed to prevent the deepening of these inequities. Policymakers and healthcare providers must work to ensure that digital healthcare solutions are accessible and affordable for all, not just the tech-savvy or economically advantaged.

Furthermore, the rise of AI in healthcare poses unique ethical dilemmas. Algorithms that assist in diagnosing conditions or recommending treatments must be transparent in their operations.

Biases inherent in AI systems, often derived from biased data or flawed coding, can lead to discriminatory practices. It is crucial to ensure that AI in healthcare operates with transparency and accountability, with checks in place to prevent perpetuating systemic biases.

As strange as it sounds, Informed consent is another critical consideration. Patients must be fully aware of how digital tools and platforms work, what data is being collected, and how it is being used.

The complexity of digital systems often makes it difficult for patients to understand these processes, thus complicating the notion of informed consent. Simplifying language, improving digital literacy, and fostering an environment of collaboration and trust between patients and providers can help mitigate this challenge.

Moreover, the human element in healthcare remains irreplaceable. While digital tools can enhance diagnostic accuracy and treatment efficiency, they should not replace human judgment and empathy.

The care provided by healthcare professionals involves a level of understanding and compassion that machines cannot replicate. The ethical approach to digital healthcare should involve integrating technology to augment human capabilities, rather than replace them.

The ethical implications of digital healthcare are not limited to the patient-provider relationship.

They extend to the broader healthcare ecosystem, including how digital tools are developed, regulated, and implemented. Collaboration between technology companies, policymakers, ethical committees, and healthcare professionals is essential to establish ethical guidelines that safeguard patient interests.

Let's not forget, As we continue to push the boundaries of what's possible with digital healthcare, ethical considerations must remain at the forefront.

Innovation should aim to enhance human well-being, prioritizing the dignity, rights, and autonomy of every individual involved. Building an ethically sound digital healthcare system requires balancing innovation with responsibility.

Education and ongoing dialogue play crucial roles in addressing ethical concerns.

Encouraging continuous professional development for healthcare providers and awareness programs for the public can foster a culture of ethical consciousness. Stakeholders must engage in open discussions to navigate the evolving ethical landscape, incorporating diverse perspectives and experiences.

International cooperation also has an important role in shaping the ethical guidelines for digital healthcare.

Different countries have unique cultural, social, and legal contexts, meaning ethical standards may vary. By sharing knowledge and experiences internationally, countries can align their efforts towards establishing robust ethical frameworks, learning from each other's successes and challenges.

To be honest, As digital healthcare continues to evolve, so too must our ethical understanding and practices.

We find ourselves at a pivotal moment, where the decisions we make today will shape the healthcare landscape of the future. By placing ethics at the core of this digital transformation, we can ensure that the future of healthcare is not only innovative but also equitable, compassionate, and just.

In conclusion, navigating the ethical terrain of digital healthcare demands vigilance, collaboration, and a commitment to protecting the fundamental rights of patients.

As we leverage technology's power to heal and enhance, we must remain steadfast in upholding ethical standards that prioritize human dignity and justice. In doing so, we can create a digital healthcare system that truly serves humanity in its entirety, ensuring that innovation leads to an equitable and brighter future for all.

Chapter 15: Cybersecurity Challenges in Healthcare

The digital landscape in healthcare is a dynamic ecosystem, teeming with innovation and cutting-edge technology poised to revolutionize patient care.

As healthcare systems transition into this digital frontier, the efficiency, connectivity, and potential of telemedicine, electronic health records (EHR), and AI-driven diagnostics promise tremendous advancements. However, these capabilities run parallel with substantial cybersecurity challenges that threaten not only data integrity but also patient privacy and safety.

The Threat Landscape

Healthcare is uniquely vulnerable to cyber-attacks due to the high value of medical data.

Personal health information (PHI) is often more lucrative on the black market than financial information because it provides a complete package of personal, financial, and medical data that is both difficult to change and permanently identifies individuals. Cybercriminals and malicious actors target healthcare institutions with increasing frequency as a result.

The rise of ransomware attacks, where criminals encrypt a healthcare organization's data and demand payment for its return, poses a critical threat.

Health systems, desperate to restore operations crucial to patient care, may be pressured into paying ransoms. This vulnerability was underscored by the infamous WannaCry attack in 2017, which afflicted numerous hospitals worldwide, leading to cancelled appointments and chaotic disruptions.

Beyond ransomware, phishing continues to be a persistent threat.

With social engineering tactics becoming more sophisticated, healthcare personnel can unknowingly provide access to sensitive information. Phishing attacks exploit human error, tricking individuals into divulging usernames, passwords, or even financial details.

Legislative and Compliance Pressures

Underpinning these cybersecurity threats is an evolving landscape of regulatory requirements.

The Health Insurance Portability and Accountability Act (HIPAA) in the United States mandates stringent measures to protect patient information. Organizations must ensure they comply with these regulations or face hefty penalties and reputational damage.

Moreover, the General Data Protection Regulation (GDPR) in Europe has set a global precedent for data protection, compelling healthcare organizations to reassess their data governance.

Non-compliance with such regulations not only affects financial stability but also erodes patient trust—the very foundation of healthcare services.

The Complexity of Legacy Systems

Many healthcare institutions grapple with the intricate challenge of legacy systems—outdated technology infrastructure that is difficult to update and secure.

These systems, often essential to day-to-day operations, can't easily integrate with modern security measures, thus providing weak entry points for cyber attackers. Migrating to newer systems poses its own set of challenges, including cost, training, and temporary disruptions to critical services.

The challenge is to balance the continued reliance on these systems while gradually integrating advanced cybersecurity solutions.

This balancing act is crucial, as outright replacement might be impractical or impossible due to budgetary constraints.

The Role of Advanced Technologies

Amid these challenges, the potential for advanced technologies to fortify defenses is promising.

Artificial intelligence and machine learning can enhance cybersecurity measures significantly. These technologies can identify patterns indicative of potential threats and detect anomalies in real-time, providing proactive measures against breaches.

Blockchain technology also presents exciting possibilities for healthcare cybersecurity.

The decentralization and immutability of blockchain provide a means of securely managing patient records and transactions, reducing the risk of data tampering. Although still in its infancy within the healthcare sector, blockchain's potential as a security measure is immense, and pilot programs are beginning to explore its applications.

Building a Cybersecurity Culture

Beyond technology, establishing a culture of cybersecurity is imperative. This involves promoting awareness and accountability at all levels of a healthcare organization.

Employees are often the first line of defense against cyber threats. Regular training sessions and simulations can help staff recognize phishing attempts, understand security protocols, and respond appropriately to potential breaches.

Moreover, fostering a collaborative culture between IT departments and healthcare practitioners is essential.

Frontline staff must be engaged in cybersecurity discussions and initiatives, as their hands-on experience provides valuable insights into potential vulnerabilities.

The Human Factor

Amid all these discussions, it's crucial not to lose sight of the human factor—the patients whose data and lives are at stake.

As we navigate the complexities of digital healthcare, patient engagement becomes a key component. Educating patients about their role in safeguarding their information, understanding the technology they interact with, and ensuring transparency about how their data is utilized builds trust and encourages participatory security.

In a world rife with cyber threats, patients deserve to feel that their data is handled with the utmost care.

Healthcare organizations must aim to balance technological advancements with ethical responsibilities, ensuring that progress does not outstrip patient security.

Looking Ahead

As we look to the future, it is clear that cybersecurity will play an increasingly pivotal role in the digital healthcare ecosystem.

This demands a proactive, multi-faceted approach—one that embraces innovation in security technologies, adheres to rigorous compliance standards, and cultivates a culture of vigilance and collaboration.

Emerging trends and technologies promise to redefine the boundaries of what is possible in healthcare security.

However, the commitment to safeguarding patient information must remain steadfast. By tackling these cybersecurity challenges head-on, we provide the foundation for a safer, more secure digital healthcare system that empowers caregivers and instills confidence in patients worldwide.

At first glance, Navigating the future requires not just technological proficiency but a resilient and resourceful mindset.

It is a journey of innovation tempered with caution—a delicate balance that ensures digital healthcare thrives amid an evolving cyber landscape.

Chapter 16: Bridging the Digital Divide

In the rapidly evolving landscape of digital healthcare, the term "digital divide" emerges as both a challenge and an opportunity. As we embrace groundbreaking technologies that redefine how healthcare is accessed and delivered, we must also confront the disparities in access to these innovations.

The digital divide represents the gap between those who have ready access to digital tools and the internet and those who do not. Addressing this divide is critical to ensuring equitable healthcare for all.

In examining the digital divide, the first step is understanding its multifaceted nature. The divide is not merely a separation between those with internet access and those without.

It encompasses a range of issues including technological literacy, geographic availability, socio-economic barriers, and cultural perceptions of digital tools. A rural community in the American Midwest might struggle with broadband accessibility, while an urban enclave in an emerging nation might face bandwidth issues due to infrastructural limitations. Simultaneously, considerations of accessibility for individuals with disabilities must be at the forefront of any comprehensive digital strategy.

Technological Literacy and Education

The journey to bridge the digital divide starts with education. It's not enough to provide the tools; we must ensure the capability to use them efficiently.

Technological literacy is fundamental in this endeavor. Educational programs tailored to various demographics, from young students to senior citizens, have shown promise in enhancing digital proficiency. Schools, community centers, and healthcare institutions can collaborate to offer workshops and training sessions that demystify digital tools.

Consider the scenario of an elderly patient who, due to mobility issues, benefits tremendously from telehealth services. However, without the knowledge to navigate the complexities of a virtual platform, the technology becomes inaccessible.

Herein lies the opportunity for educational initiatives focused on simplifying interfaces, providing straightforward instructions, and offering live support from tech-savvy volunteers. Establishing a culture of digital learning will pave the way for a future where no individual is left behind due to a lack of knowledge.

Infrastructure Investment and Development

At the heart of the digital divide is the question of infrastructure.

Many regions across the globe still lack reliable access to high-speed internet, which is a prerequisite for digital healthcare solutions. Policy makers and private corporations play an essential role in laying the physical and technological foundations necessary for digital inclusion.

Investments in infrastructure must include both macro and micro-level strategies. On a larger scale, governments can incentivize broadband expansion into underserved areas, encouraging service providers to reach out to lower-density populations.

Meanwhile, community-based initiatives can focus on establishing internet hubs and public Wi-Fi accessibility in local centers like libraries and clinics. The goal is to ensure that digital healthcare is as ubiquitous and reliable as traditional healthcare.

Economic Barriers and Collaborative Solutions

Economics also play a central role in the digital divide. High costs associated with digital devices and recurring internet service fees can be prohibitive for low-income households.

Healthcare systems and tech companies must innovate pricing models that allow for broader participation. Offering subsidized rates, creating flexible payment plans, or providing older, but functional technologies at a reduced cost are practical solutions.

Public-private partnerships can be instrumental in this regard. The synergy between governmental agencies, healthcare institutions, and tech companies can result in programs that lower the financial hurdles facing many families.

A successful example could be partnerships where tech firms donate refurbished devices to clinics in low-income areas, while governments provide tax incentives to participating companies. These collaborative efforts not only democratize digital access but also foster community solidarity.

Cultural Perceptions and Trust-building

Trust remains a pivotal element in overcoming the digital divide.

In many communities, skepticism about the efficacy and security of digital healthcare solutions can deter engagement. These perceptions are often grounded in experiences or cultural narratives that emphasize personal, face-to-face interaction over virtual interfaces.

Building trust requires culturally sensitive outreach and transparent communication. Healthcare institutions must engage with local leaders and influencers to champion the benefits of digital healthcare.

Testimonials from satisfied users, tailored communication strategies that respect cultural nuances, and privacy-focused policies are crucial in fostering trust. When patients feel secure and confident in using these digital platforms, adoption rates naturally rise.

Innovation and the Future Landscape

As we look to the future, innovation holds the key to bridging the digital divide in healthcare.

Emerging technologies such as mobile health applications designed to function efficiently on low-bandwidth networks or devices that integrate seamlessly with existing infrastructure are transformative. The development of platforms that use artificial intelligence to streamline the user experience can also reduce technological intimidation for first-time users.

Moreover, leveraging data analytics can help identify the specific needs and challenges of various communities.

Tailoring healthcare solutions based on localized data ensures that efforts to bridge the digital divide are as effective and targeted as possible.

Conclusion: Towards Digital Inclusivity

The journey toward bridging the digital divide in digital healthcare is complex yet full of potential.

It calls for a concerted effort from every stakeholder involved, including governments, healthcare providers, tech companies, educators, and the communities themselves. As we stride towards an era where technology touches every aspect of healthcare, our collective vision must prioritize inclusivity and equity.

Ultimately, bridging the digital divide is about more than just providing access; it's about empowerment. It's about ensuring that everyone, regardless of their circumstances, can engage with and benefit from the advancements in digital healthcare.

In doing so, we not only create a healthier world but also a more just and equitable one. As we continue to innovate, the digital divide can become a bridge, connecting diverse populations to a unified tapestry of healthcare possibilities.

Chapter 17: Policy and Regulation in Digital Health

In the 21st century, as digital healthcare evolves at a breakneck pace, policy and regulation stand as both the gatekeepers and enablers of innovation.

This chapter explores the intricate framework that governs digital health, focusing on the delicate balance between fostering technological innovation and ensuring safety, privacy, and equity.

The digital health revolution is reshaping the landscape of medicine, spanning telehealth, mobile health apps, wearable devices, electronic health records, and even artificial intelligence-powered diagnostics.

In this rapidly evolving ecosystem, regulatory bodies face a daunting task: crafting policies that keep pace with innovation while safeguarding patients' rights and health outcomes.

The Role of Policy in Digital Health

Policies serve as the backbone for integrating digital technologies into healthcare.

They define the standards of operation, outlining who can provide services, who bears accountability, and how data is managed and protected. As we embrace these technological advancements, policy must evolve to support a healthcare system that is accessible, affordable, and safe.

Fostering Innovation with Regulation

The speed at which technologies like AI and blockchain have permeated healthcare necessitates a regulatory framework that is not just reactive but proactive. Policies should not stifle innovation; instead, they should provide a fertile ground for breakthroughs while ensuring public safety.

An innovative approach is the concept of "regulatory sandboxes" — environments where companies can test innovative solutions within a regulatory-bound framework. These sandboxes allow for experimental implementations, providing real-world data before full-scale deployment.

In the United States, agencies like the Food and Drug Administration (FDA) are at the forefront, adapting existing frameworks to accommodate digital innovations.

The establishment of the Digital Health Innovation Action Plan and the ongoing refinement of software as a medical device (SaMD) guidelines are clear demonstrations of this adaptive regulatory approach.

Ensuring Data Privacy and Security

As the backbone of digital health, data presents unique challenges, particularly in privacy and security. With the increasing use of wearable devices and health applications, personal health information (PHI) has become more vulnerable to breaches.

Policies like the Health Insurance Portability and Accountability Act (HIPAA) set strict guidelines to protect patient data in healthcare settings. However, as technology evolves, these policies are continually challenged to cover new territories like cloud computing, AI, and cross-border health data flows.

The European Union's General Data Protection Regulation (GDPR) offers a robust model, emphasizing user consent, data minimization, and the right to be forgotten.

Its principles are increasingly being adopted globally, ensuring that patient data is treated with utmost confidentiality, thus building trust in digital platforms.

Equity and Accessibility

Digital health has the potential to democratize healthcare, providing access to remote and underserved populations.

However, without thoughtful policy intervention, there's a risk of exacerbating existing disparities. Policies must ensure equitable access to digital health services and technologies, addressing barriers such as internet access, digital literacy, and affordability.

Governments and organizations must develop strategies ensuring that marginalized populations can leverage digital health.

This includes investing in infrastructure, offering digitally-empowered education, and providing subsidies for digital health tools.

Intellectual Property and Innovation

At first glance, At the heart of digital health innovation is intellectual property (IP). Policies that protect IP rights empower companies and researchers to invest in new technology development.

However, they also run the risk of creating monopolies that can hinder accessibility. Striking a balance between protecting innovators and ensuring broad access to innovations is critical. Mechanisms like compulsory licensing and patent pools can offer solutions, promoting both innovation and accessibility.

Global Harmonization of Digital Health Regulations

In our interconnected world, digital health is a global matter. The inconsistency of regulations across borders poses a significant challenge.

Harmonizing policies could streamline processes, reduce costs, and accelerate the availability of new technologies. The World Health Organization (WHO) and other global bodies are pivotal in these efforts, working towards universal standards and facilitating cross-border innovation and cooperation.

Navigating the Policy Labyrinth

For startups and established companies entering the digital health market, navigating the complex regulatory landscape is crucial. Understanding the intricacies of regional and international laws — from the FDA in the U.

S. to the Medicines and Healthcare products Regulatory Agency (MHRA) in the UK, and similar entities worldwide — can define a company's success or failure.

Companies are encouraged to engage with regulatory bodies early in the development process.

Regular dialogue can preemptively address potential roadblocks and allow companies to integrate regulatory considerations into their product lifecycle, thus averting costly revisions or product withdrawals later.

The Future of Policy in Digital Health

As we look to the future, policy and regulation in digital health must remain agile.

Emerging technologies, such as quantum computing and advanced bioinformatics, will continue to challenge existing frameworks. Therefore, regulations must not only keep pace but also anticipate future developments.

Policy Innovation for a Health-Forward Future

It's worth noting that Embracing an innovative mindset, policymakers must develop adaptive frameworks that are as dynamic as the technologies they regulate.

Collaboration is key — between governments, the private sector, and the public. An ecosystem where innovation thrives without compromising safety, privacy, and equity is achievable.

In conclusion, policy and regulation form the pillars of digital health, built to support a future where technology and healthcare coexist in harmony.

As digital healthcare continues to evolve, strong yet flexible policies will ensure that this transformation translates into a healthier, more empowered society. The journey may be complex, but with informed, forward-thinking regulations, the potential for positive change is limitless.

Chapter 18: The Impact on Traditional Healthcare Systems

In the past two decades, our world has rapidly transformed, especially in how we access and deliver healthcare.

Digital technology, like a gentle tide that shapes the coastline, is reshaping traditional healthcare systems. In this chapter, we explore this evolving landscape where the virtual meets the tangible, examining how these changes impact patients, providers, and institutions.

The rise of digital healthcare technologies has introduced a paradigm shift, challenging the very foundations of conventional healthcare models.

Telemedicine, health apps, wearable devices, and data analytics are not mere supplements to existing healthcare systems—they are increasingly becoming integral components. The question is no longer whether digital health will impact traditional systems, but how best to integrate these technologies to enhance service delivery, improve patient outcomes, and optimize operational efficiency.

Many people don't realize this, but One of the most significant impacts of digital technology on traditional healthcare is the democratization of access. Once, healthcare was a privilege limited to those living near medical facilities, or for those who could afford to travel.

Today, telemedicine breaks these geographical barriers, bringing medical expertise to even the remotest corners of the globe. This access is particularly revolutionary in developing nations where healthcare infrastructure is sparse.

For patients, the convenience of virtual consultations is unparalleled. No longer must they endure the stress of travel or extended waiting room delays.

Instead, they can consult their physicians through video calls, secure messaging, or asynchronous platforms that allow them to submit queries or diagnostic data. This not only saves time but also minimizes the disruption of their daily lives, leading to greater patient satisfaction and adherence to medical advice.

While patients embrace these changes, healthcare providers face a dichotomy of opportunity and challenge. On one hand, digital healthcare expands their reach, allowing them to care for more patients without the constraints of physical space.

On the other hand, it demands the acquisition of new skills and adaptability to evolving technologies. Physicians and other healthcare workers must now be as fluent in technology as they are in human biology.

At first glance, Moreover, the digitization of healthcare necessitates a shift in medical education.

Institutions training the next generation of healthcare professionals must now incorporate IT skills, data interpretation, and digital ethics into their curricula. This preparation is essential, not only for the effective use of digital tools but also for ensuring patient safety and privacy in the digital age.

Healthcare institutions, much like large ships navigating a blue ocean, find themselves amid a transformation that demands agility and foresight.

Adopting electronic health records (EHRs), implementing advanced telehealth services, and leveraging artificial intelligence for diagnostics and predictive analytics are no longer optional endeavors. These technologies promise efficiency improvements—streamlining administrative processes and reducing human error—but they come with an inherent need for substantial investment, both financial and organizational.

To support this technological metamorphosis, many institutions are turning to public-private partnerships, leveraging expertise and resources outside traditional healthcare providers.

Collaborations with tech companies, start-ups, and even academic institutions enable the healthcare sector to keep pace with technological advancements. However, these partnerships also raise questions about data privacy, ownership, and the balance of power between stakeholders.

Believe it or not, Beyond the logistical and operational implications, digital healthcare is reshaping the very nature of the patient-doctor relationship. Traditionally, this relationship has been the cornerstone of medical practice, built on trust and personal interaction.

Virtual healthcare redefines this dynamic, shifting it towards a more collaborative model where patients have more control over their health data and can participate actively in their care decisions. Patients armed with information from digital sources often bring a different set of expectations to consultations, demanding more involvement in their treatment plans.

Yet, this empowerment comes with the necessity for discernment.

Not all digital health information is accurate or appropriate, requiring both patients and healthcare providers to develop digital literacy skills. Providers must guide patients through the vast seas of information online, helping them distinguish reliable sources from dubious ones.

The traditional healthcare system must also address the digital divide—ensuring that technological advancements do not exacerbate existing inequities in healthcare access.

While technology can bring healthcare to underserved populations, it requires connectivity and digital literacy, which are not universally available. Strategies to bridge this divide include investing in infrastructure, providing digital tools, and offering education and support to those previously left out of the digital realm.

Let's not forget, Finally, legal and regulatory frameworks need to adapt to the new digital landscape.

Protecting patient confidentiality and data security is paramount as more health data is stored and transmitted electronically. Regulations must evolve to ensure that digital health practices comply with ethical standards and preserve the core values of healthcare.

In conclusion, the impact of digital technology on traditional healthcare systems is multifaceted and profound. It promises to improve access, enhance efficiency, and empower patients, but it also requires us to navigate carefully to mitigate potential risks.

As we sail into the future of healthcare, collaboration, innovation, and a steadfast commitment to patient-centered care will be our guiding stars. By embracing these principles, we can harness the immense potential of digital healthcare, ensuring it serves as a beacon of hope and healing in the 21st century.

Chapter 19: Future Innovations in Digital Healthcare

In recent years, the trajectory of digital healthcare has been nothing short of revolutionary. As we stand on the cusp of unparalleled innovation, the horizon reveals a landscape poised for seismic shifts that promise to redefine the future of medicine.

At the intersection of technology and healthcare lies potential – a future where patient care is more personalized, efficient, and accessible than ever before. This chapter embarks on an exploration of this unfolding frontier, delving into the cutting-edge innovations that are set to transform the very essence of healthcare delivery.

The rise of artificial intelligence (AI) in medicine signals a fundamental change in how we approach diagnosis and treatment. AI algorithms have increasingly demonstrated their ability to analyze complex datasets with a precision that surpasses human capability. While AI's predecessor, machine learning, was limited by necessity to large, structured datasets, AI now processes unstructured data, such as electronic health records and imaging scans, to identify patterns and correlations that elude human detection.

This advancement heralds a new era of predictive analytics in healthcare. Imagine a world where a simple blood test, processed through AI, could predict the onset of diseases such as diabetes or cancer years before conventional diagnostics. This preemptive approach not only revolutionizes treatment but fundamentally alters the prevention paradigm.

Let's not forget, Yet, AI is merely the tip of the technological iceberg. Virtual reality (VR) and augmented reality (AR) are reshaping medical education and patient care. Surgeons, for instance, now use VR simulations to rehearse complex surgeries, honing their skills in an immersive, risk-free environment.

Beyond training, AR assists in live surgeries, overlaying critical information directly onto the surgeon's field of view. This transformation allows for unprecedented precision and adaptability. Patient rehabilitation, too, benefits from these technologies. Tailored VR programs help stroke patients regain motor skills, providing immersive exercises that engage the brain in ways traditional therapies cannot.

The democratization of healthcare is further realized through telemedicine, a field that has grown exponentially, particularly in the wake of global events that have emphasized the need for remote healthcare solutions. While it began as a means of alleviating geographical barriers, telemedicine now incorporates sophisticated diagnostic tools.

Smart devices, such as wearables and home monitoring kits, continuously collect health metrics, allowing for remote patient monitoring. This real-time data transmission enables healthcare providers to make informed decisions without the need for in-person consultations.

Blockchain technology, often associated with cryptocurrency, finds novel applications in healthcare. Its decentralized and immutable nature makes it ideal for handling sensitive medical data, ensuring privacy and integrity.

Blockchain technology facilitates secure patient data sharing across different platforms and institutions, paving the way for truly integrated healthcare systems. Patients wield more control over their data, selectively sharing it with providers, thus promoting a more transparent and collaborative ecosystem.

Furthermore, the synthesis of nanotechnology with digital health promises innovations at the molecular level.

Nanorobots, though nascent, offer tantalizing prospects such as targeted drug delivery, where these microscopic engineers navigate the bloodstream to deliver medication precisely where needed. This precision minimizes side effects and enhances treatment efficacy, ushering in a new epoch of personalized medicine.

Genomics and advanced biotechnologies intersect with digital health in groundbreaking ways.

The declining cost of genome sequencing means that personalized genomic data can be readily integrated into one's healthcare profile. AI-driven genomic analysis can predict how a patient might respond to certain medications, allowing for tailored drug prescriptions that reduce adverse effects and improve outcomes.

Amid these transformative technologies, the human element remains paramount. Digital healthcare innovations must always center on patient needs and ethical considerations.

As technology renders the world increasingly interconnected, digital disparities have come to the forefront. Future innovations in digital healthcare must strive to bridge these divides, ensuring equitable access to these advancements. Initiatives that expand internet access and digital literacy become vital, preventing a future where the digital healthcare divide exacerbates existing inequities.

To be honest, Data security and privacy remain of utmost concern as healthcare becomes increasingly digitized. The vast amounts of sensitive information require robust protection against cyber threats.

Innovations in cybersecurity, using AI to predict and mitigate attacks before they compromise sensitive data, are critical. Ethical guidelines must evolve alongside technology, ensuring patient rights and autonomy are preserved even as data sharing becomes more ubiquitous.

In conclusion, the future of digital healthcare is a tapestry of extraordinary innovations that promise to fundamentally transform the medical field. From AI-enhanced diagnostics to immersive training environments, from nanotechnology-driven treatments to blockchain-protected data, each advancement moves us closer to a future where healthcare is more precise, personalized, and accessible than ever before.

As we navigate this evolving landscape, our collective challenge lies in wielding these tools ethically and equitably, ensuring that this brave new world of digital healthcare enhances the human condition for all. With vigilant transparency, inclusivity, and stewardship, the innovations discussed in this chapter will forge a path to a healthier tomorrow.

Chapter 20: Conclusion: Preparing for a Digital Health Revolution

As we stand at the cusp of a digital health revolution, the possibilities appear boundless, unveiling new paradigms in how we approach wellness, patient care, and medical logistics.

Digital healthcare is no longer a futuristic vision but an imminent reality that promises to reshape the fabric of global health systems. This transformation compels us to prepare, adapt, and envision a future where technology doesn't just augment medical practices but actively revolutionizes them.

To prepare for this revolution, we must first acknowledge the democratization of healthcare. Technology has the unparalleled ability to dismantle geographical, economic, and social barriers previously inherent to healthcare access.

Telemedicine, mobile health applications, and wearable technologies have created avenues where patients can connect with professionals and health resources seamlessly and instantaneously. This ease of access empowers individuals to take health into their own hands, while simultaneously distributing knowledge and removing the monopoly held by traditional medical gatekeepers.

Interestingly enough, The empowerment of both patients and professionals is central to the digital health era. For patients, this means embracing personal health data as both a right and a responsibility. Individuals will soon rely on device-generated metrics to monitor and make informed decisions about their daily health routines.

Such data influx demands new educational efforts so users can interpret and act upon this information meaningfully. For healthcare professionals, this means adapting to a new role as interpreters and mediators of data, requiring training in digital literacy alongside traditional medical expertise. The digital health revolution will necessitate a shift from paternalistic healthcare models towards collaborative and participatory frameworks.

Equally important is the need to create an enduring foundation of trust and privacy. As health data becomes more digitized, it becomes crucial to implement robust security measures ensuring that information remains confidential and secure.

Blockchain technology's decentralized nature suggests a potential avenue for data integrity and transparency. These digital frameworks must adhere to ethical standards that prioritize patient consent and data sovereignty, building systems that protect individual privacy without stifling innovation.

Furthermore, the integration of artificial intelligence (AI) in healthcare is inevitable. AI's potential to revolutionize diagnostics, treatment algorithms, and predictive analytics is enormous, but it requires a balancing act between human oversight and machine efficiency.

Educational and regulatory systems need to evolve concurrently, ensuring that AI complements human insight rather than replaces it. As AI becomes commonplace, continuous evaluation and contextual understanding will be central to maintaining the humanity and empathy in healthcare.

It's essential to recognize the holistic potential of digital health in transcending traditional healthcare delivery, weaving into the very fabric of public health infrastructure. This revolution implores government and policymakers to adopt a proactive stance, fostering environments where innovation is encouraged and supported.

Policies must be formulated to eliminate digital disparities, ensuring equal opportunity for all sectors of the population to benefit from technological advancements. Governments have a unique role in fostering public-private partnerships, which can ignite rapid advancements and broader implementation of digital health solutions.

The trajectory of digital healthcare also demands that we address mental health with urgency and compassion.

The rise in connected devices and constant data stream places us on the precipice of an era where mental health care is increasingly digitized, offering scalable, immediate interventions. Yet, digital mental health requires careful consideration to retain the depth of human interaction intrinsic to therapeutic progress.

Moreover, the environmental impact of healthcare cannot be overlooked, as the digital health revolution presents opportunities to reduce carbon footprints by minimizing physical travel, optimizing resource allocation, and refining supply chains through predictive analytics and AI.

The digital policies we construct today must consider sustainability, integrating eco-conscious practices as a core element of development and expansion strategies.

Finally, the narrative of this revolution is predicated on the spirit of inclusivity. While an abundance of tech solutions are emerging, their deployment ought not to remain concentrated within high-income regions.

Global solidarity should guide the distribution of technology. Empowering under-resourced communities with these tools will unlock transformative potentials, reducing inequity on a worldwide scale. Embracing diversity in technological development can catalyze innovation, drawing on varied experiences to address multifaceted health challenges.

In conclusion, the digital health revolution, marked by its ambition and transformative potential, summons us to become active participants in shaping its course. It awaits us, demanding preparation grounded in education, trust, equity, and collaboration.

As we navigate this new landscape, we must envision a future where technology enhances the human experience in healthcare, rather than eclipses it, ensuring that at its core remains the unwavering commitment to improving human lives. It is not simply about the adoption of new tools, but about fostering a paradigm shift—a movement towards a healthier, more connected, and more equitable world. So let us welcome this revolution, arms open, minds ready, and hearts steadfast, as we step confidently into the dawning era of digital health.

About the Author

T. S. AVINI is a writer who believes in the power of sharing life's lessons. Having faced hardship and pain, he turned to writing as a form of self-expression and healing. Today, he pours his heart into every book, aiming to help others navigate their own struggles and find strength in vulnerability.

www.ingramcontent.com/pod-product-compliance
Lightning Source LLC
LaVergne TN
LVHW050748061126
851857LV00013B/1052
* 9 7 9 1 2 5 7 8 2 8 7 9 0 *